LET'S MAKE A PACT!

Five Ways African Americans Can Work
Together to Prevent Suicide

S. Andrea Greene

Paperback ISBN: 9798865270584
Hardcover ISBN: 9798865373841

Library of Congress Control Number: 2023920694

Book cover design by Owais Ashraf

https://www.soulsurvivors.net/

Dedication

I dedicate this book to Leon, who is gone too soon, but always remembered. May our tragedy become someone else's second chance, triumph, and helping hand when they need it most.

Table of Contents

Dear Friends,

Historically, we as a people have found strength in the warm embrace of community, and this is still true. It is within the collective heartbeat of our caring coteries that we discover the power to heal, to support, and to uplift. In the pages of this book, I invite you to join and commit, not just as individuals, but as a united force, as we work to eradicate a destructive force that decimates families as it remains shrouded in silence and stigma: suicide.

As African Americans, we embody the essence of resilience and courage. Yet, the specter of suicide has touched many lives, breaching our strong community and familial barriers. It is, in my view, a difficult conversation, but one we must have openly, compassionately, and without judgment. This book is a start, as well as a statement to our shared commitment to preventing the loss of precious lives to suicide within our community.

Just as our fingers come together to form a hand, our efforts, too, must intertwine to create a proactive, life-saving support network.

To truly comprehend the urgency of our pact, let's first look at the stark reality of suicide within our community. The statistics are not just numbers; they represent lives, dreams, and untold potential lost. In the United States, African Americans, across different age groups, are confronted with the profound impact of suicide.

According to the Department of Health and Human Services Office of Minority Health, suicide was the third leading cause of death for African American Youth, ages 15-24 (minorityhealth.hhs.gov/mental-and-behavioral-health-african-americans). This data confirms a grim reality; Every year, an alarming number of teenagers and young adults within our community experience the unbearable pain that leads to fatal, irrevocable, self-harm.

For African American adults, ages 25-54, the suicide rate has been rising steadily over the past decade, according to the National Institutes of Health. Economic challenges, systemic disparities, the effects of the pandemic, including loss of loved ones and feelings of isolation, intersect with mental health stigma and limited access to care, creating a complex landscape where individuals often endure their struggles in silence.

In our older population, suicide rates are comparatively lower, but they still exist, and are often linked to isolation, health issues, and loss.

My goal in sharing these statistics is not to instill fear but rather to ignite a fire within us. My purpose is to create a call to action, a reminder that we have the power to reverse these devastating trends. By coming together, educating ourselves, fostering understanding, and offering support, we can create a safety net that helps to ensure no one among us is left to feel alone and overwhelmed by their struggles.

As we continue our exploration of the pages that follow, let's hold onto the knowledge that together, we can make a difference. Each word read, each conversation started, and each hand extended in support is a step toward a future where the pain of suicide can be replaced by the warmth of community, understanding, and hope.

With heartfelt sincerity,

S. Andrea Greene

A Message of Hope to Anyone Who Has Lost a Loved One to Suicide

To everyone who has felt the indescribable pain that follows losing a loved one to suicide, I wrote this book with you in mind and on my heart, hoping that our collective grief can morphe into action that saves lives.

To anyone who is battling depression, mental illness, or suicidal thoughts, or you suspect your loved one may be in danger of self-harm, I have been where you are and I am here to offer hope in the form of actionable steps you can take to advance our life-saving mission.

Too many of us bear the scars of having lost a loved one to suicide. It is the dreaded club whose selection process feels random, brutal and, certainly, unwanted. Still, thousands more join, heartbroken and confused, every day, year after year.

Like you, I found myself faced with the tragic loss of a loved one to suicide, dealing with all of the complexities that accompany this type of loss, and trying to build my life anew, as the abrupt and irreversible absence of my husband meant I could not simply put the old life back together again. It just wasn't an option.

Thanks to God, a loving family, supportive community, therapy and a personal resolve, I have found purpose and joy. Now that I have reached a point in my healing journey where my cup is again filled, I am determined to pour out to others in need, and by doing so, turn my tragedy into someone else's opportunity for healing.

I see our community as fingers on a hand. Our functions are individual, but serve a collective purpose. We are interdependent on one another to achieve optimal success.

This life, our life, in this country is not always easy. It is fraught with challenges but it has also imbued us with a remarkable resilience, a spirit that refuses to be broken even in the face of unimaginable grief and loss. The pain that follows the loss of a loved one to suicide is indescribable, a profound ache that sears the soul. It's a pain that unites us, that binds us together in a shared understanding of the darkness that can cloud the mind and heart.

Yet, within this shared pain lies the spark of hope, the flicker of a candle in the midst of the deepest night. It is a hope born from the collective grief we carry, a hope that transforms our mourning into a powerful force for change. This book is not just a collection of words; it is a testament to our resilience, a manifestation of our shared determination to turn grief into action. It is a beacon of hope, lighting the way for those who are battling for their health, and even their life; it is a reminder to them that they are not alone, that there is a community standing with arms open wide, ready to embrace them.

To those who are in the midst of this battle, who feel the weight of depression, mental illness, or suicidal thoughts pressing down, I offer you not just sympathy but empathy. I have stood where you stand; I have felt the suffocating darkness that threatens to consume everything. But I have also experienced the power of hope, and discovered the strength that comes from seeking help and reaching out to others.

In this book, you will find achievable steps and practical tools that can guide you towards healing. Please remember, we are not powerless in the face of these challenges. Together, we can dismantle the stigma surrounding mental health. We can create a network of support so strong that it becomes a lifeline for those in need. We can educate, advocate, and elevate the conversation about mental health, helping to ensure that no one is left to suffer in silence.

Yes, our community is like fingers on a hand, each finger with its unique function, yet all interconnected, all essential to the collective purpose. We are not isolated individuals; we are a part of something much larger, a tapestry of lives woven together by shared experiences. And just as a hand is stronger when all its fingers work in harmony, our community becomes stronger when we unite in our mission to save lives.

Traveling this journey is not an easy task. The road is strewn with obstacles and challenges that sometimes feel insurmountable. But within these challenges lies our opportunity for growth, for resilience, for transformation. Let us not be defined by our scars but by the strength it takes to heal them. Let us turn our pain into purpose, our grief into action, and our collective commitment into hope that can guide others towards the light.

Together, we can rewrite the narrative. We can turn tragedy into triumph, despair into hope, and loss into a legacy of healing. This is our shared mission, our collective commitment, and with unwavering determination and boundless compassion, we can make a difference.

Chapter 1

Our Pact: Five Components

In the heart of our community, there lies a strength that transcends the individual—a collective power that emerges when hands join, fingers intertwine, and spirits unite. Just as the fingers of a hand work harmoniously, each with its unique purpose, essential to the whole, so too can we, as a community, come together to address a pressing concern: preventing suicide. Our unity is our greatest asset, and within it, we discover the blueprint for saving lives.

Imagine our community as a hand, outstretched and ready to offer support. Within this hand are five fingers, each representing a vital aspect of our shared commitment to suicide prevention. These fingers are more than just digits; they are the fundamental principles that embody our determination, our empathy, and our unwavering resolve. Let's examine these fingers, the foundational components of our pact, and understand how, like the fingers of a hand, they are unique yet interconnected, forming a powerful tool for change.

Education and Awareness: The Index Finger

Just as the index finger points the way, education and awareness are our guides. This finger signifies our commitment to understanding the signs, the causes, and the impact of suicide in our community. By gaining this knowledge, we dispel myths and eradicate stigma, illuminating the path toward prevention, and saving lives.

Suicide, an often unspoken and deeply stigmatized topic, lives and grows in the shadows of our collective understanding. That is why actively raising awareness is our lantern, providing light that pierces through the darkness which surrounds and provides cover to this existential issue. It's about breaking the silence, breaking the stigma, and breaking down the walls that prevent honest conversations about mental health.

Through community workshops, social media campaigns, and grassroots initiatives, we can shine a spotlight on the realities of suicide.

By intentionally bringing the conversation into the public sphere, we normalize discussions around mental health struggles and suicidal ideation. Through our discourse, we can share stories of survival and resilience, emphasizing that seeking help is not a sign of weakness but a testament to one's strength.

In our awareness-raising endeavors, we can target not only those directly affected but the broader community. We need to engage schools, workplaces, and community centers, creating an environment where mental health is a priority that requires attention, instead of a taboo subject to be avoided.

Another way to raise awareness is through the integration of mental health education into curriculums and workplace programs. By doing so, we equip individuals with the knowledge they need to identify signs of distress and offer support.

Media also plays a pivotal role. Responsible portrayal of mental health struggles in movies, TV shows, and accuracy in reporting helps dispel harmful stereotypes and provide a more accurate understanding of the complex factors contributing to suicidal ideations and attempts at self-harm. Celebrities and public figures openly sharing their mental health journeys can amplify the message, and thankfully, this is occurring more often. Their stories help drive home the reality that, regardless of our status or background, mental wellness can be a struggle.

Collaboration with mental health professionals, educators, and policymakers is essential. By working hand in hand, we can develop comprehensive awareness campaigns tailored to different demographics and appealing to diversity within and across cultures. These campaigns not only highlight the prevalence of suicide but also emphasize the availability of resources and support networks.

Online platforms can serve as powerful tools for raising awareness. Social media campaigns, webinars, and podcasts reach vast audiences, sparking conversations that might not otherwise occur. Online support groups provide safe spaces for individuals to share their struggles, fostering a sense of belonging and reducing the isolation that often accompanies suicidal thoughts. More people need to know that these spaces exist.

By collectively illuminating the dark corners of suicide, we create a culture where seeking help is not just encouraged but expected. Through our ongoing efforts, we work toward building a society where no one feels alone in their battle against mental health challenges.

Imagine you have a superpower – the ability to understand the unspoken words hidden behind someone's smile or subtle changes in their behavior. This superpower is not magical or imaginary. It is the language of care, a skill we all can cultivate to support our loved ones.

Every person we know speaks a silent language that tells us how they feel without uttering a word. It is in the sudden or incremental withdrawal from activities they once loved, change in sleep patterns, or the persistent sadness clouding their eyes that words are spoken. These are sometimes not just ordinary behaviors; they may be signals, whispers from the heart telling us something is wrong. Unfortunately, these unspoken words and signals are not always heard or noticed.

When someone is struggling mentally or emotionally, it is common for their behavior to undergo changes. These changes can be subtle or blatant. For example, some people might become unusually irritable, withdraw from social activities, or neglect personal hygiene. Others may engage in risk-taking behaviors, begin to give away cherished belongings or talk in code, giving instructions to loved ones on what to do if something happens to them. These changes are not just coincidences; they are signs, indicating an inner battle.

The saying, "words have power" is true, and when someone is contemplating suicide, they might drop hints. Phrases like "I can't take it anymore" or "I wish I weren't here" could be cries for help. Pay attention, not just to what they say, but how they say it – the tone, the hesitation – these nuances matter. Let the person you know you have heard them by probing. Do not simply allow such statements to go unanswered. For example, you might respond by asking, "You wish you weren't where?" or "What can't you take"? You can offer a lifeline by acknowledging their frustration or despair and asking how you can help.

Now, imagine emotions as waves – usually, they have gentle ebbs and flows. But when someone is struggling, these waves can turn into tumultuous storms. Sudden mood swings, from extreme sadness to uncharacteristic bursts of anger, can signify an emotional turbulence that needs our understanding and attention.

Consider this: Have you noticed someone pulling away from friends and family, retreating into solitude? Social isolation, although common, can be a red flag, potentially indicating feelings of hopelessness and despair. The best way to find out if someone you care about is in trouble is to reach out - even if they seem reluctant. This especially includes your so-called strong family, friends and associates. They sometimes need help the most, and are the least likely to ask for it. Your presence might be the lifeline they need.

Sleep disturbances may also be a warning sign. These disturbances might seem mundane and unimportant on the surface, but they can be indicators of significant distress. Whichever extreme, insomnia, oversleeping, loss of appetite, or sudden overeating can all be signs that someone is struggling to cope. Gentle probing and keen observation are your best tools to offer concern and support to someone who may be struggling with feelings of despair.

Speaking of despair, when someone expresses feelings of hopelessness or a belief that things will never get better, it is more than just negativity; it is a cry for help. These expressions of despair are the language of care, urging us to extend our hands in support.

When someone uses terms like never and forever in the contexts of hopelessness or despair, they are attaching permanence to a situation, circumstance or feeling that is subject to change over time. Some things we can do to help include offering perspective and support. Remind the person that even the most difficult circumstances can and do change for the better in time. Offer your presence, knowledge and resources, reassuring your loved one that you are committed to aiding them in their wellness. Remember, understanding the language of care doesn't require special training – it requires empathy, patience, and the willingness to listen. By honing our ability to recognize these signs, we can become not just observers but active participants in someone's well-being. Let's be vigilant, let's be compassionate, and let's be the caring community that saves lives, one conversation at a time.

I see knowledge as a sturdy bridge that connects us to a world of understanding and compassion. In the realm of mental health and suicide prevention, this bridge is our lantern of hope. It's not just about facts and figures; it's about arming ourselves with the understanding needed to make a difference, not only in our lives but in the lives of those around us.

The first step toward empowerment is understanding mental health. It is not a distant, abstract concept as some believe; it is a vital part of our overall well-being. It is also important to note that mental health challenges are not character flaws; they are real, psychological conditions that affect countless individuals. Religion and cultural perceptions have incorrectly led many of us to misjudge the nature of mental illness, to the detriment of many in the community. However, when we grasp the truth about the actual root causes of mental illness, we can eradicate the judgment and stigma that have clouded our understanding of mental health and mental illness for far too long.

Knowledge equips us with the ability to recognize the signs of emotional distress in others. When we understand that sudden behavioral changes, verbal cues, or expressions of hopelessness can be indicators of someone's existential struggle, we can become vigilant guardians of their well-being. When we are armed with knowledge, we are equipped to step into the realm of active empathy, offering a compassionate listening ear, even when we are unable to understand someone else's plight.

Another benefit of gaining knowledge is it guides us to resources. From hotlines to community support groups, therapy, and counseling services, these resources can become lifelines for individuals in crisis. Once we know how to access services, we can become connectors, linking people to the help they need. We can also become advocates, ensuring that help is always within reach.

Education bridges gaps in understanding. When we educate ourselves, we become bridges in our communities, opening conversations that were previously taboo. By sharing what we know, we dismantle myths and replace ignorance with understanding. We become catalysts for change, transforming our communities into places where mental health is a priority and compassionate support is readily available.

As we grow in knowledge, we are likely to also become more empathetic, and empathy in action equals support. When we understand the journey of recovery and healing, the importance of patience, and the power of non-judgmental encouragement, we become pillars upon which someone can lean. Our knowledge guides us to offer more than sympathy. Genuine empathy enables us to shine a light of hope during someone's darkest hours.

In this shared pursuit of understanding and knowledge through education, we empower ourselves and others. We become advocates, educators, and compassionate listeners. By gaining knowledge, we develop the power to change lives, to offer solace, and to be the unwavering support that someone needs.

Supportive Communities: The Middle Finger

I submit, the preventive middle finger serves a useful purpose, unlike the negative connotation often attached to this digit. It stands tall, the same way in which supportive communities provide strength and stability.

This metaphorical finger symbolizes our dedication to creating safe spaces where individuals can share their struggles without judgment. In communities with a strong middle finger, empathy and understanding reign, fostering an environment where healing meets encouragement.

Think of a lighthouse, guiding ships safely to shore. Our communities, too, can be like lighthouses, providing a steady light and direction toward solid ground in the face of life's tempests. The middle finger, much like the lighthouse, represents the stability and strength of supportive communities in the realm of suicide prevention.

In our communities there exists a circle of compassion, a historical bond of kinship and shared experiences, a space where empathy knows no bounds. It is within this circle that we can find the strength to face life's challenges, including the difficult battle against suicidal thoughts. Supportive communities are not just safety nets; they are foundations upon which individuals can rebuild their lives.

So, if not supportive communities, consider the alternative: isolation, which can create a deafening echo of negative inner thoughts, distorting reality and magnifying the pain of those battling mental health issues. A proactively supportive community is the best weapon in the war against loneliness and isolation.

Belonging is a fundamental human need, and supportive communities offer a sense of unity and belonging that is unparalleled. They are places where individuals are not defined by their struggles but by their resilience. Within these communities, people find kindred spirits, forging connections that provide solace and the courage to face each new day. Connection is the antidote to despair, and supportive communities facilitate these vital connections. Be it through support groups, online forums, or community events, these spaces foster bonds that promote healing. In the embrace of a supportive community, individuals find respite, gain perspective, and discover the strength to continue their journey toward recovery.

Finally, imagine our community as a single, collective heartbeat – steady, strong, and filled with hope. This heartbeat resonates within supportive communities, nurturing hope in the hearts of those who feel hopeless. A place where stories of triumph over adversity are shared, replacing hopelessness with hope.

Supportive communities are more than gatherings of individuals; they are living, breathing organisms of empathy and understanding. Each member is a vital thread, weaving a tapestry of hope that blankets the entire community. Together, in the embrace of these communities, we find the strength to

face the darkest of times and emerge
stronger, united, and filled with the promise of
a brighter tomorrow.

Access to Mental Health Care: The Ring Finger

The ring finger represents commitment, and ensuring access to mental health care for all is a commitment to overall well-being.

This finger underscores our resolve to break down the barriers that prevent individuals from accessing the care they need. It signifies our advocacy for affordable, culturally competent mental health services in every community, regardless of socioeconomic status, educational background, employment status or any of the other artificial barriers that currently exist.

In the realm of mental health care, access is the most vital component. Without it, even the most advanced, efficient health care system is useless and failing the people it is supposed to serve. Picture this: someone facing the depths of despair, longing for a lifeline, a glimmer of hope. Access to mental health services is that lifeline, a bridge between anguish and healing. It is not a luxury; it is a fundamental right, regardless of a person's background or circumstances.

Yet, this lifeline often hangs out of reach for far too many. Economic disparities and systemic barriers create a gap, leaving individuals stranded in their struggles. But here's the thing: this gap is not insurmountable. It is a challenge we, as a community, can overcome together. To overcome the access obstacle, advocacy must become our tool, our collective voice demanding equality in access. By standing up, by making our voices heard, we can continue to push for policies that ensure mental health services are not a privilege but a right for all.

Now, let's imagine a world where seeking therapy doesn't involve navigating bureaucracy and financial hurdles, where mental health services are as accessible as a neighborhood clinic (though I realize neighborhood clinics are not always accessible, either). This vision need not be a far-off dream; it is a reality we can create.

Community-driven initiatives and awareness campaigns can bridge this gap, offering guidance on navigating the system and connecting individuals with the help they need.

Additionally, cultural competence in mental health care is not a bonus; it is a necessity. Picture someone, already vulnerable, seeking help and encountering professionals who understand their language and their unique cultural context. The result can be transformative. Culturally competent mental health care is the key to breaking down barriers of understanding, ensuring that every individual, regardless of their cultural background, feels seen, heard, and supported on their journey to healing.

In this pursuit of accessible and culturally competent mental health care, education becomes our ally. By informing our communities about their rights, available resources, and how to navigate the system, we empower individuals to advocate for themselves. Education is not just knowledge; it is the pathway to empowerment, a torch illuminating the way toward accessible mental health care for everyone.

Cultural Competence and Sensitivity: The Little Finger

Just as the little finger is often underestimated, the necessity of cultural competence in healthcare is often overlooked.

The little finger emphasizes the importance of mental health professionals who understand our unique cultural backgrounds. It signifies our demand for respectful, sensitive care that acknowledges and appreciates our community's diversity. It is also a metaphor, reminding us that the things that appear to be small, matter.

Now, imagine the importance of cultural competence in mental health care as a delicate thread, weaving its way through the fabric of support. Just as the little finger plays a significant role in the hand's intricate tasks, cultural competence ensures that mental health services are tailored to fit the diverse needs of our community. It's not just about understanding different languages; it's about comprehending the nuances of traditions, beliefs, and values that shape an individual's perspective.

In mental health care, these nuances matter profoundly. Picture someone grappling with anxiety, seeking solace in therapy. Now, imagine their relief when the therapist not only speaks their language but also understands the cultural context, acknowledging the interplay of heritage and mental health. It is more than comfort; it is validation, a feeling that one's identity is respected and understood.

Culturally sensitive mental health care can be powerful in its efficacy. It bridges gaps in understanding, shortens the distance between professional and patient and builds trust. When mental health professionals embrace cultural competence, they are able to offer more than therapy; they can provide a sanctuary in which individuals can express their struggles without fear of misjudgment, where every aspect of their identity is acknowledged and valued.

Cultural competence is not an add-on; it is a fundamental element that ensures mental health services can resonate throughout our diverse community. We need to create therapeutic spaces where individuals feel seen and heard. When individuals receive care that aligns with their cultural background, it is akin to the little finger finding its perfect place in the hand – a harmonious fit that makes the entire system stronger and more effective.

In our pursuit of mental health support, let's champion the cause of cultural competence. Let's advocate for training programs that instill cultural sensitivity in mental health professionals. Let's celebrate the richness of our community's diversity, ensuring that everyone, regardless of their cultural background, receives care that recognizes their uniqueness.

Breaking the Stigma: The Thumb

The thumb supports at a distance, closing the gap and bridging barriers, similar to the way we continue to work to break the stigma surrounding mental health.

This finger demonstrates our determination to challenge societal norms and transform attitudes toward mental health. It signifies our unwavering resolve to replace judgment with understanding, eliminating shame as a barrier to seeking help.

Consider the thumb in the context of mental health advocacy. Much like the thumb supports and enables a wide range of hand movements, breaking the stigma surrounding mental health supports a multitude of potentially life-changing conversations. This act of breaking barriers is not just about challenging societal norms; it's about dismantling the preconceived notions that have kept mental health conversations in the shadows, often with devastating consequences.

Imagine someone, burdened by depression, feeling the weight of societal judgment press down upon them. Now, picture the impact when the thumb, symbolizing the breaking of stigma, intervenes. It pushes back against judgment, allowing individuals to share their stories without shame or fear. Breaking the stigma is not just a symbolic gesture; it is a revolutionary act that transforms societal perceptions, turning ignorance into understanding and exclusion into acceptance.

Breaking the stigma is about an entire community embracing the idea that mental health is as important as physical health. It entails understanding that mental health challenges can affect anyone, regardless of age, gender, or background. When we break the stigma, we create an environment where individuals do more than talk about mental health; they openly discuss their struggles, their triumphs, and their journey toward healing.

Consider a world where no one feels hesitant to seek therapy, where discussing therapy is as normal as talking about a visit to the dentist. This world, free from the chains of stigma, is not unachievable; it can be a reality within our grasp. When we open the floodgates of conversation, allowing empathy to flow freely, the voices of judgment and ignorance are silenced.

In our everyday interactions, let's challenge misconceptions and myths about mental health. Let us be the thumb that pushes back against stigma, embracing those who feel alienated and isolated. Let's celebrate the courage of those who share their mental health journeys, making it clear that seeking help is not just acceptable; it's commendable. Together, as a community, let's reshape the narrative around mental health, creating a space where the thumb, in its symbolic gesture, becomes a powerful force, paving the way for acceptance, understanding, and compassion.

Chapter 2

Stories of Resilience and Hope

It's true, too many of us share the unalterable experience of losing a loved one to suicide. One is too many lives lost, too many loved ones impacted, and it happens more often than you might think. The weight of our individual and collective sorrow, at times, seems unbearable, immeasurable. Yet, in the heart of our shared experiences, sometimes hidden among the stories of loss and pain, there exists a collection of narratives that echo with the profound strength of the human spirit. This chapter opens a door into the deeply personal and profoundly courageous journeys of individuals who have faced the daunting specter of mental health challenges and the devastating aftermath of loss.

These stories are more than ink on paper; they are living chronicles of endurance, illuminating the often arduous path from darkness to light. Within these pages, you will find tales of remarkable individuals who, through their unwavering resolve, have transformed pain into power and despair into determination. Each story is a testament to the resilience that resides within us all, exhibiting the incredible capacity of the human heart to overcome adversity.

These narratives are more than anecdotes; they are beacons of hope illuminating the way for others who might be navigating similar struggles. Through the raw honesty of these stories, we find solace in the shared human experience, understanding that we are not alone in our battles. They remind us that amidst life's trials, there exists a wellspring of hope, urging us to reach out, to support one another, and to believe in the possibility of healing.

As we immerse ourselves in these stories, let us approach them not merely as accounts of hardship, but as sagas of resilience, strength, and, above all, hope. May these stories serve as a source of inspiration, reminding us of the extraordinary power we possess to rise above challenges and emerge stronger on the other side. Through these narratives, we reaffirm our collective commitment to fostering a community where compassion thrives, understanding flourishes, and hope becomes the guiding light, leading us all towards brighter tomorrows.

My Story

I will begin with my own personal story. I was
about 22 years old. My daughter was two, and
my son was just a year old. I was young,
single, mom, struggling in multiple areas of my
life. Just a few years earlier, I was a bright
high school student, with a future filled with
promise, a debutante with dreams of attending
Howard University. But, things changed during
my senior year of high school. My focus
shifted, my grades plummeted and, instead of
going to Howard, I enlisted in the Air Force.
Mind you, serving our nation will always be an
honorable undertaking and the Air Force is the
elite of all service branches, but it was vastly
different from the path I imagined I would take.

While waiting for the date I was scheduled to
attend basic training, I worked, went to the
local junior college and… met a guy and fell in
love. Nothing unusual about an 18-year-old
falling in love, right? Well, somehow, the test
that was administered right before I went to
Lackland didn't detect I was pregnant. Now
that was unusual.

Anyway, during basic training, I noticed I was gaining weight, always sleepy and experiencing cravings. I didn't get alarmed until I reached tech school. By then, three months had passed since I left the small town I graduated from to go off into the world in a way I believed would allow me to exert my independence. With more free time, and more weight gain, I decided to visit the clinic on base. Once I explained my symptoms to the doctor, she asked, "When was the last time you had a period?" I replied, "I haven't been sexually active for three months. She replied, "Let's take a test just to be sure. Call the office in three days for the results."

Three days later, right after class, I called the office as instructed and was informed the test result was positive. Completely naive, I asked, "Positive means I'm not pregnant, right"? Go ahead and laugh. I was young. I still laugh at myself every time I think about it. When the voice on the line replied, "No ma'am, it means you are," I did not know what to think or how to feel. I purchased several rolls of quarters and called the young man I had been calling and writing for months to tell him we were having a baby. We used all the quarters that day and ultimately decided he would come where I was. Once he arrived and we were faced with the prospect of becoming parents at 19, love began to transform into abuse and pain.

Fast forward, an early but honorable discharge, a baby girl, a baby boy and 3 years later…Young love had died, and I was alone with two children (whom I loved dearly) to raise, no sense of direction, no job, and no support from the children's father. This was not what I had imagined. Most days, I focused on taking care of my children, building my family and I was still holding on to hope with the father. One day, I don't remember exactly what disappointment or pressure was the trigger, but I became overwhelmed with sadness.

I remember the pain I was feeling that night in the darkness of our duplex apartment. I sat the kids on the living room couch, went into the kitchen and removed a knife from the drawer. I returned to the living room and kneeled on the floor in front of the chair that was near the couch and began to cut my left wrist. The knife that I used to cut everything else hardly broke the skin. I looked over at my small children, not saying a word, but looking at me. I began to sob. Still on my knees, I cried out loud, "I don't want to die. I just don't want to live like this." I stopped cutting and called my mother. Her voice was more stern than normal when she said, "Grab your kids right now, get in your car and come here." I did exactly as she asked. She lived about 20 minutes away by car. I don't remember what happened when I arrived at her house. I don't remember if we talked about what led me to harm myself. We did not discuss things like that back then, so it's safe to assume we did not. Instead, we kept going. A couple scars from the cuts I made remained on my wrist for years as a reminder. I never intentionally cut myself again.

I am certain my mother helped me save my own life that night. I do not think about or wonder what would have happened had she not answered the phone, or if she had failed to grasp the seriousness of the situation. I do occasionally see my children's faces in my mind as they were that night, and I am so thankful we were all given a second chance for a better outcome, together.

My daughter and son are now 32 and 31, and I have a two-year-old granddaughter who I completely adore and spoil! Today, I am so grateful I had the presence of mind to notice my children watching, and to admit the truth about what I was feeling (I didn't want to die. I just wanted my life to change.). I am grateful that I called my mother and for her stern advice. Today, I am sure there was love in her counsel. Today, I am grateful that I lived to earn three degrees, including a Masters. My life did change. I am grateful for a strong sense of purpose and for a journey that has taught me to love myself, that life ebbs and flows and it is during our hardest times that our character is built and lasting lessons are learned. Today, I am grateful that I survived to raise my family, to do what I love and help others overcome their struggles. I am grateful that I did not make a decision that would have permanent consequences for so many over a temporary circumstance.

It has taken years for me to embrace my entire life's story. But, through education, retrospection, experience and a commitment to self-love, I have learned that a painful chapter, a disappointing event or even a devastating tragedy are not signs that life is over, but opportunities to grow, to become wiser and stronger. They are the rain before the rainbow, and although they usually don't feel good, they can still be used to do a good work in us.

NOTE: If you or someone you love is struggling with suicidal thoughts, help is available. Dial 911 or call 988 to reach the Suicide and Crisis Lifeline. For online support, findahelpline.com has a list of resources available 24 hours a day, 7 days a week.

Maya's Story

While many stories end tragically, thankfully, there are many that have a positive outcome. Maya's story is one that gives us hope. Let's take a look.

Maya was a big city girl with a big smile. But, behind her radiant smile, Maya carried a heavy burden – a burden that seemed insurmountable at times. She battled with profound sadness and an overwhelming sense of hopelessness, feelings that pushed her to the edge of despair. One fateful night, these feelings grew unbearable, and she found herself standing on the edge of a bridge, contemplating a tragic decision.

As fate would have it, Officer Daniels, a compassionate police officer on patrol that night, spotted Maya and sensed her despair. With a heart full of empathy, he approached her cautiously, his voice gentle yet firm. "I can't imagine the pain you're feeling, but I know there's help available. Can we talk?" he asked, his eyes reflecting genuine concern.

At that moment, something stirred within Maya. A flicker of hope, however faint, ignited. She agreed to talk, and Officer Daniels, recognizing the urgency of the situation, connected her with a crisis helpline. On the other end of the line was Sarah, a mental health professional trained to handle such delicate situations. With a soothing voice, she listened as Maya poured out her heart, her pain, and her fears.

Sarah, understanding the critical nature of the situation, immediately coordinated with a nearby mental health facility that offered 24/7 crisis intervention. Maya was gently guided there, where she was met with a team of empathetic psychologists and counselors. In those moments, she found the help she desperately needed.

Maya's journey toward healing had just begun. With access to mental health care, she received therapy tailored to her needs, medications to stabilize her emotions, and most importantly, a support network that surrounded her with understanding and compassion. The therapists, counselors, and support groups became her pillars of strength, helping her navigate the tumultuous waters of her emotions.

Over weeks and months, Maya's resilience shone brightly. With therapy and the unwavering support of her mental health care team, she learned coping mechanisms, rebuilt her self-worth, and discovered a newfound hope for life. Her journey was not easy, but every step forward was a victory, a testament to the power of accessible mental health care and the strength of the human spirit.

Maya's story became a ray of hope within her community. It highlighted not only the importance of intervention but also the significance of accessible mental health care. Her experience underscored the critical role that easy access to professional help plays in saving lives. Maya's story became a driving force in her community's commitment to the pact, reminding everyone that with the right support, even in the darkest of times, there is hope.

Andre's Story

In a small town nestled between rolling hills, lived a young man named Andre. Behind his charismatic smile and outgoing demeanor, Andre hid a secret burden: a profound battle with anxiety and depression that left him feeling isolated and desperate. The stigma around mental health in his community weighed heavily on his shoulders, making him hesitant to reach out for help.

One evening, as his thoughts grew darker, Andre decided he couldn't bear the pain any longer. He composed a heartbreaking farewell letter, ready to end his struggle. Just as he was about to take that tragic step, his phone buzzed with a message. It was from his childhood friend, Gary, who sensed something was wrong from his recent social media posts.

Fearful for his friend's safety, Gary trusted his instincts and rushed to Andre's house. Finding the farewell letter, he immediately pleaded with him, "Andre, please don't do this. Your life matters. Let's fight this battle together." Gary reminded Andre that it is ok to struggle and need not pretend to be ok when he isn't. It is not uncommon for African American men to feel uncomfortable talking about their struggles and expressing their emotions. Thankfully, Gary was caring enough to give Andre permission to be honest without fear of judgment.

Thanks to Gary's genuine concern and commitment, something shifted inside Andre. He felt a glimmer of hope, a tiny crack in the darkness that had enveloped him. He put down the pills he had planned to take, and instead, he opened up to Gary about his struggles. For the first time, he spoke openly about his feelings of despair, fear, and hopelessness.

Gary, understanding the weight of the stigma surrounding mental health, knew that Andre needed more than just his support. He encouraged Andre to speak to his family and friends about his struggles, breaking the silence that had kept him captive. In time, they both initiated conversations within their community, challenging the misconceptions about mental health and urging others to share their stories without shame.

As more people opened up about their own battles, the community began to embrace a new narrative—one of empathy, understanding, and support. Mental health awareness events were organized, where survivors shared their stories of resilience, and mental health professionals debunked myths about therapy and treatment.

In this atmosphere of openness and acceptance, Andre found the courage to attend therapy. His therapist, well-versed in the nuances of breaking the stigma, provided a safe space where Andre could discuss his feelings without judgment. With therapy and the unwavering support of his community, Andre gradually emerged from the depths of his despair.

With time, Andre's perspective shifted. He realized that his mental health challenges did not define him; they were a part of his story, but not the whole story. Empowered by his journey, he became an advocate, sharing his experiences at local schools and community centers, offering hope to others who felt trapped by the stigma.

Andre's story became a testament to the transformative power of breaking the silence around mental health. It showed his community that by embracing openness and understanding, lives could be saved.

Leila's Story

In a vibrant multicultural neighborhood lived a woman named Leila, whose smile masked a silent battle with depression. Her cultural background made it challenging for her to open up about her struggles; the fear of being misunderstood in the predominantly non-native community amplified her pain. It seemed like a bleak and solitary journey until she met Dr. Patel, a mental health professional renowned for his cultural competence and sensitivity.

One day, Leila, overwhelmed by her emotions, walked into Dr. Patel's clinic, her heart heavy with despair. Dr. Patel, recognizing the importance of cultural sensitivity, greeted her warmly, speaking her native language fluently and understanding the intricacies of her cultural context. Leila, for the first time, felt truly heard and understood.

In their sessions, Dr. Patel created an environment of trust and acceptance. He delved into more than Leila's symptoms; he examined the cultural nuances that influenced

Leila's mental health. Through patient listening and empathetic understanding, he deciphered the unspoken fears and anxieties that had burdened her for years.

Dr. Patel's approach was holistic. He incorporated elements from Leila's cultural background into her therapy, integrating traditional healing practices and rituals that held significance for her. This amalgamation of culturally competent therapy made Leila feel acknowledged and empowered her to confront her challenges with newfound strength.

As weeks turned into months, Leila's resilience grew. With the guidance of Dr. Patel, she learned coping mechanisms rooted in her cultural beliefs, dismantled the barriers of stigma within her community, and found the courage to engage with her support network. Her family, initially hesitant to discuss mental health, began attending sessions with her and learned how to support her effectively.

With time, Leila's mental health improved dramatically. She not only found relief from her depression but also became an advocate within her community, breaking the silence surrounding mental health issues. Dr. Patel's cultural competence did more than save Leila's life; it had transformed it, allowing her to reconnect with her cultural heritage and find strength in her identity.

Leila's story highlights the immense impact of culturally sensitive mental health care, showing that understanding an individual's cultural background is not just a gesture of respect but a lifeline. Through the competence and sensitivity of mental health professionals like Dr. Patel, lives can be transformed, stigma shattered, and communities can begin to heal, one empowered individual at a time.

In the pages of this chapter we journeyed through personal narratives that vividly demonstrate the significance of the pact and its pivotal components. These stories, whether centered around the importance of presence and reaching out, accessing mental health care, breaking the stigma, or fostering cultural competence, showcase the transformative power of empathy, understanding, and support. They underline the importance of the pact's components in real, tangible ways, depicting how accessible mental health care can be a lifeline, how breaking the silence can save lives, and how cultural competence can bridge gaps of understanding. Through these narratives, the pact emerges as a set of principles as well as a living, breathing testament to the potential of human compassion. These stories emphasize that in embracing the pact, we forge pathways toward healing, offer refuge to the distressed, and ultimately, weave a tapestry of hope and resilience within our communities.

Chapter 3

The Role of Allies and Advocates

In the sphere of mental health support, allies and advocates stand as the unsung heroes, the steadfast pillars upon which individuals in crisis lean. This chapter delves into the profound impact these compassionate souls have on the journey of mental health, in and outside the community. Here, we explore the stories of those who, out of empathy and understanding, have become champions of change. Their unwavering dedication to breaking the stigma, fostering inclusivity, and providing unyielding support paints a portrait of hope and resilience. This chapter is a testament to the extraordinary power of empathy, illustrating how each ally and advocate is a candle on a hill, illuminating the path for others to follow. I am so glad you are still with me, forging ahead in discovering how we can make an "im-PACT"! The goal in sharing these inspiring tales is to illustrate how the extraordinary care and concern of ordinary people can lift others up in the face of mental health challenges, and to learn how their life-saving actions, both big and small, shape a future where understanding and support can become a beautiful new normal. Hopefully, you can see yourself in their stories and decide how you, too, can become a community advocate.

First, let's look at Mark's story…

In the heart of a bustling city, situated in a vibrant Black community, there was a medium –sized organization. In this workplace, change was on the horizon, thanks to Mark Thompson, an ally with a mission.

A compassionate and open-minded individual, Mark was a manager working in an environment where mental health discussions were often hushed, and stigma cast a shadow over those who needed help. Determined to make a difference, Mark embarked on a personal journey of education and understanding.

His first step was to educate himself. He spent late nights poring over books. Whenever possible, he attended seminars, and even enrolled in free, online courses focused on mental health awareness. He familiarized himself not just with the statistics but the human stories behind them. The knowledge he gained gave him the confidence to begin subtly introducing mental health topics into workplace conversations, breaking the ice with statistics. He later added personal narratives. Over time, Mark helped to normalize discussions around mental health in his workplace.

It wasn't long before spearheading conversations turned into advocacy. With approval from senior leadership, he organized lunchtime sessions where experts were invited to speak about mental health. These sessions became safe spaces for employees to share their experiences, fostering a sense of camaraderie. Mark's empathetic approach and genuine interest in the well-being of his colleagues made him a trusted confidant. Slowly, the barriers of fear and ignorance began to crumble.

One day, Mark organized a mental health awareness day at the workplace. The office was transformed into an oasis of information, adorned with posters, pamphlets, and resources. He encouraged open discussions about stress, anxiety, and depression.

Colleagues, initially hesitant, found solace in sharing their stories, realizing that they were not alone in their struggles.

Mark's dedication didn't go unnoticed. Senior management, inspired by his initiative, implemented mental health support policies. They introduced counseling services, mental health days, and regular workshops focused on stress management and emotional well-being. The workplace became a center of mental health support, and it was Mark's unwavering commitment that helped to make it possible.

Over time, Mark's advocacy extended beyond the workplace. He volunteered at community events, sharing his knowledge and encouraging others to join the conversation. Mental health became a topic no longer whispered but spoken about openly, reducing the stigma that once shrouded it.

Mark's journey as an ally transformed the workplace and, by extension, the larger community. His passion, empathy, and dedication became a catalyst for change, breaking down barriers, and paving the way for a future where mental health was not just acknowledged but embraced. His story became an inspiration, a reminder to everyone that one person's advocacy could indeed change the world, one workplace at a time.

Now, let's learn about the positive impact of Kate's advocacy:

After witnessing a friend's mental health crisis, a young and spirited advocate, Kate, a teacher, found her purpose in a small, predominately white town: promoting mental health awareness beyond the boundaries of her community. Armed with determination and the power of social media, Kate set out on a mission to make a difference.

Kate began her journey by immersing herself in the world of mental health advocacy. She attended workshops, read extensively, and connected with experts. Equipped with knowledge, she turned to social media, recognizing its immense potential to create positive change.

She started a blog, "Mindful Moments," where she shared stories of hope, along with coping strategies and resources. Through insightful articles and heartfelt personal accounts, she touched the hearts of readers in her community and beyond. Her social media platforms became safe havens, where people could openly discuss mental health without fear of judgment.

Realizing the importance of early intervention, Kate turned her attention to schools. She collaborated with other educators, creating engaging online content tailored for students. Animated videos, interactive quizzes, and live Q&A sessions became her tools to educate young minds about mental health. Through virtual sessions, she encouraged dialogue, teaching students that seeking help was a sign of strength, not weakness.

Kate's influence extended to workplaces as well. She partnered with companies to conduct online workshops on stress management, mindfulness, and creating mental health-friendly workplaces. Her webinars, live streams, and social media campaigns reached employees across diverse industries, fostering a culture of understanding and support.

But Kate didn't stop there. She initiated online challenges and campaigns, urging people to share their mental health stories using specific hashtags. The internet buzzed with personal accounts of triumph over adversity, inspiring others to speak up and seek help. Her campaigns went viral, reaching millions, and encouraging communities to have open conversations about mental health.

One of her most impactful initiatives was the creation of a mental health support app. Through crowdsourcing and collaborations, she developed a user-friendly platform that connects individuals in need with mental health professionals. The app provided a lifeline for those struggling, offering resources, helplines, and therapeutic exercises.

Kate's dedication caught the attention of influencers, celebrities, and mental health organizations. Together, they formed a digital alliance, leveraging their collective reach to amplify mental health awareness.

Through Kate's digital advocacy, the conversation around mental health transcended geographical boundaries. More schools became nurturing environments where students could discuss their feelings openly. Some workplaces transformed into spaces where employees felt valued, supported, and understood. Many communities grew in empathy, standing together to break the stigma surrounding mental health.

Kate's story spread, inspiring others to utilize social media for good. In a world often dominated by negativity, she proved that the digital realm could be a sanctuary of compassion, education, and hope. Through her efforts, Kate demonstrated that one person, armed with passion and a smartphone, could indeed make a difference, one post at a time.

Mark and Kate's stories are examples of how and why allies play a pivotal role, weaving threads of understanding and support from both within and outside the Black community.

Within, it is necessary to nurture a sense of belonging and acceptance. Allies can foster an environment where discussing mental health is encouraged and normalized. Within the Black community, allies can help break the chains of stigma that have bound mental health discussions for too long. By sharing personal stories, advocating for mental health resources, and embracing cultural competence, they create safe spaces where individuals can express their struggles without fear of judgment.

Outside the community, allies can contribute by educating themselves about the unique challenges faced by the Black population concerning mental health. Cultural sensitivity becomes paramount here. Allies can engage in conversations, not just as observers, but as active listeners. By acknowledging the historical context, systemic disparities, and the intersectionality of race and mental health, they help bridge the gap of understanding. They can advocate for equal access to mental health services, ensuring that resources are not only available but tailored to meet the diverse needs of the Black community.

Moreover, allies, both within and outside, can actively challenge stereotypes and prejudices. By questioning harmful narratives and advocating for accurate representation in the media, they can break down the barriers that prevent open conversations about mental health. Allies can also support Black-led mental health organizations, amplifying their voices and initiatives.

It is imperative that allies stand in solidarity with the community consistently, not just when a local story sparks a national discussion. They can promote mental health education in schools, workplaces, and communities, ensuring that awareness becomes an integral part of everyday conversations. By fostering a culture of empathy, allies contribute to creating an atmosphere where seeking help is viewed and treated as an act of courage.

As we have demonstrated, being an advocate means more than just raising awareness; it involves taking tangible steps to create a supportive, understanding community. Here are seven detailed, actionable steps that individuals can undertake to become effective advocates for mental health and suicide prevention:

1. Educate Yourself and Others:

Start by educating yourself about mental health issues, suicide prevention strategies, and the specific challenges faced by different communities. Once you are well-informed, share this knowledge with others. Engage in conversations, dispel myths, and promote accurate information. Knowledge is a powerful tool that can challenge stereotypes and foster empathy.

2. Destigmatize Mental Health:

Actively challenge stigma whenever you encounter it. This could mean correcting misconceptions, speaking openly about your own experiences if you feel comfortable, or engaging in campaigns that promote mental health awareness. By normalizing conversations around mental health, you contribute to a culture where seeking help is viewed as a sign of strength.

3. Support Mental Health Initiatives:

Support and volunteer with mental health organizations, hotlines, or crisis intervention services. Your time and skills can make a significant difference. By actively participating in mental health initiatives, you directly contribute to the resources available to those in need.

4. Advocate for Policy Changes:

Advocate for policies that improve mental health care accessibility, affordability, and quality. This could involve writing to local representatives, participating in advocacy campaigns, voting for candidates who support progressive mental health policies or supporting organizations that work toward mental health policy reforms. By influencing policies, you help create a more supportive environment for those struggling with mental health issues.

5. Promote Mental Health in Schools and Workplaces:

Advocate for mental health education in schools and workplaces. Encourage institutions to implement mental health programs, workshops, and support services. By fostering mental health awareness from a young age and creating supportive environments in workplaces, you contribute to prevention efforts and early intervention.

6. Be a Compassionate Listener:

Practice active listening and empathy. Sometimes, all someone needs is a listening ear. Be non-judgmental, patient, and understanding when someone opens up about their mental health struggles. Your support can make a world of difference and might encourage them to seek professional help.

7. Use Social Media for Good:

Utilize your social media platforms to share mental health resources, stories of hope, and supportive messages. Social media can be a powerful tool for spreading awareness and breaking stigma. By using your online presence positively, you reach a wide audience and contribute to changing societal attitudes.

By taking these actionable steps, you become a part of the movement to affect change in the realm of mental health and suicide prevention. Your advocacy efforts, no matter how small, contribute to creating a world where mental health is prioritized and support and resources are abundant and accessible.

Chapter 4

Coping Strategies and Self-Care

In the tapestry of African American lives, there are threads woven with strength, resilience, and a rich cultural heritage. However, it is essential to recognize that this strength does not equal immunity to stressors but rather a testament to endurance in the face of unique challenges. African Americans often confront stressors that stem from systemic inequalities, historical injustices, and societal prejudices. These stressors, interwoven with daily life, can create an intricate web of pressure that weighs heavily on mental health.

One significant misconception that permeates the community is the belief that strength means suppressing one's emotions and neglecting self-care while prioritizing the needs of others. This false perception is rooted in historical narratives of endurance against immense odds. While resilience is undoubtedly a defining trait, it is important to acknowledge that resilience doesn't entail simply enduring silently; it means confronting challenges with courage, seeking support, and nurturing one's mental and emotional well-being.

The pressure to be strong often leads individuals to ignore their feelings, burying emotions deep within themselves. This emotional suppression can lead to a detrimental cycle, where unaddressed stressors accumulate, creating an overwhelming burden. Moreover, neglecting self-care in favor of caregiving for others might seem noble, but it comes at a cost. It can lead to burnout, emotional exhaustion, and a depletion of mental and physical resources.

Acknowledging emotions and practicing self-care are not signs of weakness. They are acts of profound strength. It takes courage to confront one's vulnerabilities, to admit when the burden becomes too heavy, and to seek help. Strength lies in embracing the full spectrum of human emotions, acknowledging pain, and allowing oneself to heal.

By dismantling the misconception that strength means enduring in silence, the African American community can pave the way for open conversations about mental health. It is necessary to foster an environment where individuals feel safe to express their emotions, seek therapy without stigma, and prioritize self-care without guilt. This shift in perception doesn't diminish the community's resilience; instead, it enhances it. When individuals are emotionally supported and mentally well, they can face challenges with clarity and fortitude.

In essence, the true strength lies not in enduring alone but in reaching out, not in neglecting oneself but in nurturing one's well-being. By embracing these truths, the African American community can create a culture where mental health is prioritized, support is abundant, and the narrative of strength evolves into one of holistic well-being. This transformation not only benefits individuals but strengthens the entire community, creating a legacy of resilience rooted in self-care and emotional well-being.

In the heart of self-care is the practice of mindfulness, a timeless technique rooted in the art of being fully present. Imagine it as a gentle anchor in the stormy sea of thoughts and emotions. Mindfulness techniques, such as deep breathing exercises, invite you to embrace each breath as a moment of stillness. Inhale tranquility, exhale tension; it is a dance between your breath and the present moment. Incorporate mindful walking into your routine. Feel the earth beneath your feet with each step, grounding yourself in the present. In moments of stress, grounding exercises bring you back to reality – feel the texture of an object in your hands, listen to the sounds around you, breathe deeply. Mindfulness is not intended to silence your mind; it is about observing your thoughts without judgment. With practice, it can become a sanctuary, a space where you can find peace in the midst of the chaos.

Cognitive-behavioral techniques, often hailed as the toolkit for reframing negative thoughts, empower you to challenge the stories your mind weaves. Start by identifying negative thoughts – the 'I'm not good enough' or 'I'll never succeed' narratives. Are they rational? Challenge them. Replace 'I can't do this' with 'What can I learn from this?' By questioning your thoughts, you dismantle their power over your emotions.

Journaling can also become a powerful ally in this journey. It is not just words on paper; it is a mirror reflecting your thoughts and fears. Pour your heart out; it's a conversation with yourself, a way to unravel the complexity of your emotions. Through the act of writing, you gain clarity, allowing you to challenge negative patterns and find new perspectives.

Gratitude, a practice often underestimated, is a transformative force. Gratefulness helps you find beauty in the ordinary, and acknowledge the small moments of joy. Each day, take a moment to reflect on three things you're grateful for. They could be as simple as the sun warming your skin or the aroma of freshly brewed coffee. Gratitude shifts your focus from what's lacking to what is abundant in your life.

Positive affirmations, akin to planting seeds in the fertile soil of your mind, have the power to reshape your self-perception. Repeat affirmations daily; they could be about your worth, your strength, or your ability to overcome challenges. In these affirmations, you will find the courage to face adversity, the belief in your potential, and the strength to endure.

Physical well-being is the cornerstone upon which mental health rests. Regular exercise is about more than physical fitness; it is one component of a holistic approach to well-being. When you move your body, you release endorphins – the body's natural stress relievers. Exercise doesn't have to be intense; even a leisurely walk in nature can be therapeutic.

Nutrition is another component of well-being as it fuels not only your body but also your mind. A balanced diet rich in fruits, vegetables, whole grains, and lean proteins nourishes your brain and supports emotional well-being.

Adequate sleep is the body's way of healing and rejuvenating. Prioritize sleep; create a bedtime routine, limit screen time, and create a restful environment. In these acts of self-care, you invest in your overall health. Your body and mind are interconnected; when you nourish one, you fortify the other.

Creative expression is a language of emotions. Engage in artistic endeavors; let the colors on a canvas mirror your feelings. Art is not about perfection; it's about expression. The strokes of a brush or the movement of your hands in clay become a dialogue with your soul. Writing is a cathartic journey. Write freely, without judgment; it could be a journal entry or poetry that echoes your innermost thoughts. Music, the universal language, has the power to stir your emotions. Create playlists that resonate with your feelings – music can be a companion in your moments of solitude and a celebration in moments of joy. In these creative outlets, you find solace, a way to express what words cannot encapsulate. They become the bridge between your emotions and the external world.

Building a supportive network can be reflective of your strength, not evidence of your weaknesses, as some believe. You are not alone in this journey. Cultivate connections with friends, family, and support groups. Talk openly about your struggles; allowing yourself to be vulnerable with people you trust is a testament to your courage. Seek professional help if needed. Therapists are guides through the labyrinth of emotions. In these connections, you find understanding, compassion, and the reassurance that you are never alone. Opening up to others is not a burden; it's an act of self-care, a step toward healing.

In the embrace of these coping strategies and self-care practices, you will find tools to manage your emotions and nurture a loving relationship with yourself. As you learn to recognize your worth, honor your emotions, and acknowledge your resilience, you discover not only the strength to face challenges but also the wisdom to cherish moments of joy. Self-care isn't selfish; it is a declaration of your worthiness. Through these techniques, you cultivate an inner sanctuary, a space of compassion and acceptance. Remember, self-care is not a destination; it is a continuous journey, a sacred commitment to becoming the best version of yourself. In these practices, you find not just coping mechanisms but lifelong companions on your path to mental and emotional well-being.

Chapter 5

Our Collective Commitment

In our community, there exists a collective strength, a bond forged through shared experiences, culture, and history. Within this unit, we find our commitment – a commitment to one another, to our families, and to the generations to come. It is a commitment that transcends words, a silent vow that echoes through time, resonating with the resilience of those who have faced adversity and triumphed.

This commitment finds its embodiment in the pact we have explored, a powerful framework designed to safeguard our community from the shadows of despair. The pact, with its five components similar to the fingers of a hand, represents not just a set of principles, but a profound promise. It signifies our dedication to the well-being of our fellow community members, our willingness to break the chains of stigma, and our shared determination to foster an environment where mental health is not just valued, but prioritized.

The first component, raising awareness, is the light that illuminates the path. It signifies our commitment to shedding light in the dark crevices of mental health, dispelling myths, and encouraging open conversations. Awareness becomes the foundation upon which understanding is built, and understanding, in turn, becomes the cornerstone of empathy.

The second component, identifying risk factors and warning signs, is our language of care. It's about recognizing the silent cries for help, understanding the subtle nuances of distress, and responding with compassion. By educating ourselves and our community about these signs, we equip ourselves with the knowledge to intervene, to reach out a helping hand when someone is drowning in despair.

The third component, the power of knowledge, represents our commitment to empowering ourselves and others. Knowledge becomes our armor against ignorance, our tool to dismantle prejudices, and our bridge to understanding mental health complexities. By being informed, we break down barriers and pave the way for informed decisions and compassionate actions.

The fourth component, supportive communities, signifies our promise to be not just bystanders but active participants in each other's lives. We become beacons of support, offering solace, understanding, and a listening ear. Communities are not just safety nets; they are the foundations upon which lives are rebuilt, the hands that lift us when we stumble.

The little finger, the fifth component, represents access – access to mental health care, to therapies, and to resources. It signifies our collective commitment to tearing down barriers that prevent individuals from seeking help. Access becomes the golden thread that weaves the fabric of mental health support, ensuring that no one is left behind, that help is always within reach.

Our collective commitment is not a distant ideal; it's a promise we make in our daily interactions, in our willingness to listen, in our empathy, and in our actions. It's a commitment that transcends generations, passing on the torch of compassion and understanding to those who come after us.

As you read these words, I invite you to make your commitment to the pact. Embrace it as more than a set of principles, but as a way of life. Raise awareness in your community; educate yourself about mental health and its complexities. Be vigilant about the signs of distress, not just in others but also within yourself. Empower yourself with knowledge and extend that knowledge to others. Be a pillar of support in your community, and advocate for accessible mental health care. Let your commitment become a ripple, spreading far and wide, creating a wave of change that transforms lives.

In this collective commitment, we find the strength to face the challenges of mental health together. We become not just individuals, but a united force, a community that stands tall in the face of adversity. Let your commitment be the spark that ignites a revolution of understanding, support, and love. Together, we can create a future where mental health is a priority, where no one suffers in silence, and where every life is cherished. This commitment is not just a pledge; it's a legacy we leave for the generations to come, a testament to our collective strength and compassion.

In Closing: A Call to Action

And one final, important thing: as you close this chapter, I urge you to consider the power of connection in our commitment to mental health and suicide prevention. It's not just about understanding the principles outlined in this book; it's about putting them into action in our daily lives.

I invite you to choose someone, a friend, a family member, a colleague – someone you care about deeply – and make a pact. Agree to be there for each other, to be a shoulder to lean on in times of darkness. Promise to let them know if you're struggling, to reach out when the weight of the world feels unbearable. And equally crucial, pledge to check on them regularly, at least once a month. Ask how they're doing, inquire about their mental well-being, and truly listen to their response.

In this simple yet profound act of reaching out and staying connected, we become the safety nets for one another. We break the silence that often shrouds mental health struggles, replacing it with open conversations and genuine care. It is in these everyday gestures of kindness and concern that we truly live the principles of our commitment. Together, as individuals bound by empathy and understanding, we can create a community where no one suffers in silence, where support is abundant, and where every life is valued.

Remember, in our collective commitment, every action, no matter how small, contributes to our collective hope and healing. Let us be the change-makers, the listeners, and the advocates. By making this pact, you are no longer just a reader; you are an active participant in the transformative journey towards mental health and well-being. Let this commitment echo through your actions, inspiring others and shaping a future where compassion reigns, and no one walks the path of mental health challenges, loss, grief and pain alone.

About the Author

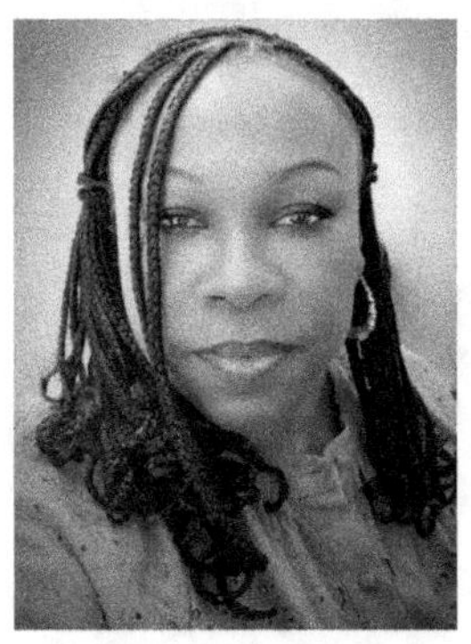

S. Andrea Greene, a compassionate, dedicated advocate for mental health and well-being, is the founder of Soul Survivors Support Services, LLC. With a Master of Science degree in Counseling Psychology, S. Andrea's journey into the realm of grief support and mental health advocacy was deeply personal.

Driven by her own profound experience of losing a loved one to suicide, S. Andrea founded Soul Survivors Support Services, LLC, a guiding light of hope and solace for those navigating the complexities of grief. With unwavering dedication, she provides essential services, offering individual and group support to widows and widowers, extending a helping hand to those affected by suicide, and providing much-needed support to loss survivors.

S. Andrea's expertise is not confined to theoretical knowledge; it is a fusion of academic acumen and heartfelt empathy. Through her organization, she has become a symbol of hope for individuals seeking solace and understanding amidst the darkness of grief. Her approach is rooted in genuine compassion, understanding, and the belief in the power of community.

In addition to her professional endeavors, S. Andrea is an advocate for suicide prevention, dedicating her efforts to raising awareness and offering support to those in crisis. Her impactful journey has transformed into a lifeline for others, a testament to the resilience of the human spirit, and a testament to the power of turning personal tragedy into an opportunity for healing and support.